Table of Contents

INTRODUCTION

Infertility is something both men and women struggle with. So, does CBD oil help or hurt your chances at pregnancy?

CBD oil has been praised for its many potential health benefits and its use in the treatment of several chronic and acute conditions. However, despite CBD oil's growing popularity, there are still a number of unanswered questions like, does CBD oil affect fertility?

Currently, there's a lack of evidence to definitely state whether CBD oil has a positive or negative effect on human fertility. While products derived from cannabis are now legalized in most states, there are ethical implications of conducting tests on individuals who are trying to become pregnant. Because of this, We might not have a conclusive answer as to whether CBD oil impacts fertility for years to come.

While using CBD oil may indirectly help with conception-related issues that aren't physical in nature (e.g. sleep and mood), there are also studies that have shown CBD oil consumption could negatively affect fertility. In short, the jury's still out on whether using CBD oil could positively or negatively affect one's ability to get pregnant, which is why it's important to do as much research as possible on CBD oil and fertility before making a final decision.

Below, we'll go over what we currently know about Infertility, CBD oil's and potential benefits and risks as they apply to human fertility. With this information, you can decide on the best path forward for you and your partner.

When you're trying to get pregnant, there's no shortage of holistic treatments that people say you should do to "boost" your fertility or increase your chances of conceiving. One of these "natural" products that people are particularly interested in for fertility purposes is cannabidiol, or CBD, the non-psychoactive compound found in cannabis and hemp.

Sound sketchy? It's wise to be somewhat skeptical about the seemingly ubiquitous compound making its way into every wellness product. Despite the lack of regulation or scientific proof that CBD does anything, many people still use the products. But if you're someone who's trying to get pregnant, you might be extra concerned about the effect that CBD could have on you and potentially your future baby.

Past research has shown that using cannabis that contains THC, the psychoactive compound that contributes to a high, is not a good idea for people who are trying to get pregnant. It has been recommends that people stop using marijuana before trying to get pregnant, because it can negatively impact the fetus's development as early as the first trimester of pregnancy. On top of that, a male partner's weed use is just as important: Studies have shown that men who use marijuana regularly have reduced sperm concentrations by 28% compared to those who don't.

While we know that cannabis can contribute to male infertility, "we do not yet know if CBD products made from cannabis might also have a negative effect," explains Julie Lamb, MD, FACOG, medical advisor at Modern Fertility. CBD is so new that there haven't been any solid studies to show that it's safe in pregnancy, or specifically what effects CBD hemp oil would have on a fetus, she adds. In one study that was conducted on mouse embryos, researchers found that the compound anandamide, which is increased with CBD use, actually inhibited the development of embryos, she says.

For all of these reasons, when a couple is having difficulty conceiving, they avoid CBD. But this also brings up an important point regardless of whether or not you're trying to conceive: it's always a good idea to check with your doctor before you try CBD. Although CBD seems harmless, the effects could interfere with other drugs or treatments. Until we know more about CBD, it's better to be safe than sorry.

And finally, just because someone suspects that CBD was able to solve all their fertility issues, that doesn't mean that the same is true for you. As we've said before, when you're trying so many different things to get pregnant, it's impossible to say what actually "worked." Even if everyone swears CBD really "works."

INFERTILITY

Infertility happens when a couple cannot conceive after having regular unprotected sex.

It may be that one partner cannot contribute to conception, or that a woman is unable to carry a pregnancy to full term. It is often defined as not conceiving after 12 months of regular sexual intercourse without the use of birth control. In the United States, around 10 percent of women aged 15 to 44 years are estimated to have difficulty conceiving or staying pregnant. Worldwide, 8 to 12 percent of couples experience fertility problems. Between 45 and 50 percent of cases are thought to stem from factors that affect the man.

Causes in men

The following are common causes of infertility in men:

Semen and sperm

Sometimes the sperm cannot travel effectively to meet the egg.

Semen is the milky fluid that a man's penis releases during orgasm. Semen consists of fluid and sperm. The fluid comes from the prostate gland, the seminal vesicle, and other sex glands.

The sperm is produced in the testicles.

When a man ejaculates and releases semen through the penis, the seminal fluid, or semen, helps transport the sperm toward the egg.

The following problems are possible:

Low sperm count: The man ejaculates a low number of sperm. A sperm count of under 15 million is considered low. Around one third of couples have difficulty conceiving due to a low sperm count.

Low sperm mobility (motility): The sperm cannot "swim" as well as they should to reach the egg.

Abnormal sperm: The sperm may have an unusual shape, making it harder to move and fertilize an egg.

If the sperm do not have the right shape, or they cannot travel rapidly and accurately towards the egg, conception may be difficult. Up to 2 percent of men are thought to have suboptimal sperm.

Abnormal semen may not be able to carry the sperm effectively.

This can result from:

A medical condition: This could be a testicular infection, cancer, or surgery.

Overheated testicles: Causes include an undescended testicle, a varicocele, or varicose vein in the scrotum, the use of saunas or hot tubs, wearing tight clothes, and working in hot environments.

Ejaculation disorders: If the ejaculatory ducts are blocked, semen may be ejaculated into the bladder

Hormonal imbalance: Hypogonadism, for example, can lead to a testosterone deficiency.

Other causes may include:

Genetic factors: A man should have an X and Y chromosome. If he has two X chromosomes and one Y chromosome, as in Klinefelter's syndrome, the testicles will develop abnormally and there will be low testosterone and a low sperm count or no sperm.

Mumps: If this occurs after puberty, inflammation of the testicles may affect sperm production.

Hypospadias: The urethral opening is under the penis, instead of its tip. This abnormality is usually surgically corrected in infancy. If the correction is not done, it may be harder for the sperm to get to the female's cervix. Hypospadias affects about 1 in every 500 newborn boys.

Cystic fibrosis: This is a chronic disease that results in the creation of a sticky mucus. This mucus mainly affects the lungs, but males may also have a missing or obstructed vas deferens. The vas deferens carries sperm from the epididymis to the ejaculatory duct and the urethra.

Radiation therapy: This can impair sperm production. The severity usually depends on how near to the testicles the radiation was aimed.

Some diseases: Conditions that are sometimes linked to lower fertility in males are anemia, Cushing's syndrome, diabetes, and thyroid disease.

Some medications increase the risk of fertility problems in men.

- ❖ Sulfasalazine: This anti-inflammatory drug can significantly lower a man's sperm count. It is often prescribed for Crohn's disease or rheumatoid arthritis. Sperm count often returns to normal after stopping the medication.
- ❖ Anabolic steroids: Popular with bodybuilders and athletes, long-term use can seriously reduce sperm count and mobility.
- ❖ Chemotherapy: Some types may significantly reduce sperm count.
- ❖ Illegal drugs: Consumption of marijuana and cocaine can lower the sperm count.
- ❖ Age: Male fertility starts to fall after 40 years.
- ❖ Exposure to chemicals: Pesticides, for example, may increase the risk.

- ❖ Excess alcohol consumption: This may lower male fertility. Moderate alcohol consumption has not been shown to lower fertility in most men, but it may affect those who already have a low sperm count.
- ❖ Overweight or obesity: This may reduce the chance of conceiving.
- ❖ Mental stress: Stress can be a factor, especially if it leads to reduced sexual activity.

Laboratory studies have suggested that long-term acetaminophen use during pregnancy may affect fertility in males by lowering testosterone production. Women are advised not to use the drug for more than one day.

Causes in women

Infertility in women can also have a range of causes.

- ❖ Smoking significantly increases your risk of infertility
- ❖ Age: The ability to conceive starts to fall around the age of 32 years.

- ❖ Smoking: Smoking significantly increases the risk of infertility in both men and women, and it may undermine the effects of fertility treatment. Smoking during pregnancy increases the chance of pregnancy loss. Passive smoking has also been linked to lower fertility.

- ❖ Alcohol: Any amount of alcohol consumption can affect the chances of conceiving.

- ❖ Being obese or overweight: This can increase the risk of infertility in women as well as men.

- ❖ Eating disorders: If an eating disorder leads to serious weight loss, fertility problems may arise.

- ❖ Diet: A lack of folic acid, iron, zinc, and vitamin B-12 can affect fertility. Women who are at risk, including those on a vegan diet, should ask the doctor about supplements.

- ❖ Exercise: Both too much and too little exercise can lead to fertility problems.

- ❖ Sexually transmitted infections (STIs): Chlamydia can damage the fallopian tubes in a woman and cause inflammation in a man's scrotum. Some other STIs may also cause infertility.

- ❖ Exposure to some chemicals: Some pesticides, herbicides, metals, such as lead, and solvents have been linked to fertility problems in both men and women. A mouse study has suggested that ingredients in some household detergents may reduce fertility.

- ❖ Mental stress: This may affect female ovulation and male sperm production and can lead to reduced sexual activity.
- ❖ Medical conditions

Some medical conditions that can affect fertility includes:

Ovulation disorders appear to be the most common cause of infertility in women.

Ovulation is the monthly release of an egg. The eggs may never be released or they may only be released in some cycles.

Ovulation disorders can be due to:

Premature ovarian failure: The ovaries stop working before the age of 40 years.

Polycystic ovary syndrome (PCOS): The ovaries function abnormally and ovulation may not occur.

Hyperprolactinemia: If prolactin levels are high, and the woman is not pregnant or breastfeeding, it may affect ovulation and fertility.

Poor egg quality: Eggs that are damaged or develop genetic abnormalities cannot sustain a pregnancy. The older a woman is, the higher the risk.

Thyroid problems: An overactive or underactive thyroid gland can lead to a hormonal imbalance.

Chronic conditions: These include AIDS or cancer.

Problems in the uterus or fallopian tubes can prevent the egg from traveling from the ovary to the uterus, or womb.

If the egg does not travel, it can be harder to conceive naturally.

Causes include:

Surgery: Pelvic surgery can sometimes cause scarring or damage to the fallopian tubes. Cervical surgery can sometimes cause scarring or shortening of the cervix. The cervix is the neck of the uterus.

Submucosal fibroids: Benign or non-cancerous tumors occur in the muscular wall of the uterus. They can interfere with implantation or block the fallopian tube, preventing sperm from fertilizing the egg. Large submucosal uterine fibroids may make the uterus' cavity bigger, increasing the distance the sperm has to travel.

Endometriosis: Cells that normally occur within the lining of the uterus start growing elsewhere in the body.

Previous sterilization treatment: In women who have chosen to have their fallopian tubes blocked, the process can be reversed, but the chances of becoming fertile again are not high.

Medications, treatments, and drugs

Some drugs can affect fertility in a woman.

Non-steroidal anti-inflammatory drugs (NSAIDs): Long-term use of aspirin or ibuprofen may make it harder to conceive.

Chemotherapy: Some chemotherapy drugs can result in ovarian failure. In some cases, this may be permanent.

Radiation therapy: If this is aimed near the reproductive organs, it can increase the risk of fertility problems.

Illegal drugs: Some women who use marijuana or cocaine may have fertility problems.

Cholesterol

One study has found that high cholesterol levels may have an impact on fertility in women.

Global CBD Exchange

So, with cannabis taking center stage as the new miracle drug, many people are wondering whether cannabis can also help increase a woman's likelihood of getting pregnant. Does it improve female fertility or does it impede it?

Cannabis and ovulation

A review of clinical literature in 2002 published in the Journal of Pharmacology found that the use of cannabis decreases the level of luteinizing hormone (LH) secreted by the pituitary gland. LH is a sex hormone that triggers the ovulation.

One of the studies cited in this review had tested the impact of THC in monkey ovulation, and it was found that LH levels dropped 50-80%, causing ovulation to stop. However, after 3 to 4 months of using THC, the monkeys started ovulating and menstruating again. This meant that as they built tolerance for THC, things returned to normal and the monkeys had no more trouble conceiving.

When it comes to fertilized ovum, time is very essential. Once an ovum is fertilized, it needs to implant onto the uterus within a certain time period before it loses its viability. And because cannabis can delay the speed by which the fertilized ovum travels, a new formed embryo may be unable to implant in time to create a viable pregnancy. This results to early miscarriage, or even to ectopic pregnancy.

There are both male and female factors to be aware of. By taking control of your fertility you can stand up to possible fertility challenges. It is important to remember that infertility challenges are very common and that there are various treatments available.

To increase chances of conception it is important to foster adequate sexual exposure, healthy eating habits and maintain a healthy weight. Factors that decrease chances of conception include stress, alcohol (abuse), smoking and recreational drug use. All of the above apply to men and women.

You don't have to see a specialist or go through expensive treatments immediately. A general practitioner will be able to guide you based on the information you provide. Factors to rule out include intercourse timing, stress, medications that could be interfering, depression/anxiety and STDs. Provided answers and applicable test results will help determine the way forward.

The Next Step for Men

The next recommended step is not invasive and produces fast results. Simply go for a semen analysis. Once a sample has been collected, the semen itself as well as the number, shape and movement of sperm it contains can be analysed.

If no abnormalities are found, there are other causes to be rule out, but there are also female factors to consider at this stage.

The Next Step for Women

Determining female infertility factors are not always as simple. Various primary care tests could be required before a condition is diagnosed and treated to allow natural conception. Challenges can include:

Ovulation problems

Blocked fallopian tubes

Menstrual irregularities

Hormonal imbalance

Post abortion damages

Recurrent miscarriage

Fibroids

There are other female-specific medical conditions that can be treated and managed to allow natural conception, however, in some cases specialist care is required to assist women who have:

Endometriosis

Pelvic adhesions

Decreased ovarian reserve

Pelvic inflammatory disease

Polycystic ovarian syndrome (PCOS)

When Infertility Challenges are Still Not Resolved

If primary care treatments are not sufficient, specialist care as well as advanced care treatments and procedures are available.

CBD OIL

CBD stands for cannabidiol. It is one of 113 cannabinoids that's found in cannabis. It is non-addictive and also non-psychoactive. CBD is extracted from the cannabis plant during production and is separated from the THC, which is the psychoactive element of cannabis. Cannabidiol (CBD) is one of many cannabinoids that can be found in hemp and marijuana, two types of cannabis plants.

CBD may help people with cancer manage some symptoms of the disease as well as side effects of treatment. Scientists are also looking into how CBD could aid cancer treatment, but more research is needed before any conclusions can be made.

Marijuana has enough tetrahydrocannabinol (THC) to get you high, but hemp does not. CBD itself has no psychoactive compounds

CBD oil has garnered a reputation as being an effective treatment for neurological and physiological illnesses. People who use CBD oil love that it's a natural product that is generally much easier on the body when compared to most pharmaceuticals. It's commonly used to treat pain, anxiety, and insomnia, but can CBD oil work for cancer patients?

Those that want to seek the supposed relief that cannabis may provide, may now seek it through the use of CBD. Those suffering from anxiety, depression, pain, cancer, and other ailments are turning to CBD for the possible relief and bodily equilibrium that it may provide. There are not any known health risks associated with CBD... however; those taking certain medication should proceed with caution. In any case, we recommend consulting with a medical professional for those who take medication which may interact with grapefruit (Read more about CBD drug interactions here. In fact, there are innumerable reports throughout common widespread media that attribute CBD to its' positive prophylactic effects

This book will take an in-depth look at everything you need to know about using CBD for cancer treatment.

How Are CBD Products Made?

Many people know that CBD comes from cannabis. It's right there in the name: cannabidiol.

But, how exactly does CBD oil get made? What happens in the transition from the hemp plant to a product you can buy online or in your local health store?

All CBD products contain CBD oil, which is extracted from the hemp plant. This is why you'll often see "hemp extract" on the label and in the ingredients list. After extraction, the oil is added to various products, including CBD oil tinctures, gummies, capsules, topicals, and vape oils.

CBD Extraction Methods

When people talk about how CBD products are made, they're mainly talking about the specific extraction method.

The most common methods to extract CBD oil use carbon dioxide, steam distillation, or hydrocarbon or natural solvents. We review each of these below.

Carbon Dioxide (CO2) Extraction

CO2 extraction uses supercritical carbon dioxide to separate the CBD oil from the plant material. "Supercritical" refers to the CO2 containing properties of both a liquid and a gas state, which is why you'll sometimes see this method referred to as Supercritical Fluid Extraction (SFE).

During CO2 extraction, a series of pressurized chambers and pumps are used to expose CO2 to high pressure and very low temperatures, resulting in an extracted oil containing high amounts of CBD.

At the start of extraction, one chamber will hold pressurized CO2, while a second pressurized chamber holds the hemp plant.

The CO2 is then pumped from the first chamber into the second. The presence of supercritical CO2 breaks down the hemp also in the chamber, causing the oil to separate from the plant material.

Finally, the CO_2 and oil are pumped together into a third chamber. The gas evaporates, leaving an extract of pure CBD oil behind.

While it requires expensive specialized machinery, CO_2 extraction is the preferred method for making CBD products. It's extremely safe and efficient at producing high concentrations of CBD in the resulting oil—as much as 92% according to one analysis.

Carbon dioxide extraction for CBD oil

The precise nature of CO_2 extraction also makes it suitable for producing specific concentrations of CBD oil. Manufacturers can simply adjust the solvent and pressure ratios to achieve the desired concentration of CBD.

The CO_2 extraction process is also widely used to create many other products besides CBD oil, such as decaffeinating coffee or tea, or extracting essential oils for use in perfumes.

Steam Distillation

With steam distillation, steam causes the CBD oil to separate from the hemp plant. The hemp plant is contained in a glass flask, with an inlet and an outlet. The inlet connects to another glass container, beneath the plant flask, that contains water that is set to boil. The outlet connects to a condenser tube. As the water heats up, the steam travels upwards into the plant flask, separating the oil vapors that contain CBD.

These vapors are then captured in a tube that condenses them into oil and water.

Once collected the oil and water mixture is distilled to extract the CBD oil from the water.

The steam distillation technique is tried and true, having been used to extract essential oil for centuries, but it's less preferred than CO2 extraction due to its inefficiency. Steam distillation requires significantly larger amounts of hemp plant, and it's more difficult to extract exact amounts of CBD concentration using this method.

There's also an element of risk with this method. If the steam gets too hot, it can damage the extract and alter the chemical properties of the cannabinoids it contains.

 Solvent Extraction (Hydrocarbons and Natural Solvents)

Solvent extraction follows a similar process to steam distillation, except that it uses a solvent rather than water to separate the CBD oil from the plant material. This creates a resulting mixture of the CBD oil with the solvent. The solvent then evaporates leaving pure CBD oil behind. Solvent extraction uses either hydrocarbons or natural solvents.

Solvent extraction is more efficient than steam distillation, and it's also less expensive. However, the solvents used in hydrocarbon extraction (including naphtha, petroleum, butane, or propane) create cause for concern. The solvent residue can be toxic and increase one's cancer risk if they aren't fully eliminated during the evaporation step—which doesn't always happen. Some studies have found traces of petroleum or naphtha hydrocarbons residue in CBD products that used solvent extraction.

To avoid the risk of toxic residue, solvent extraction can use natural solvents instead, such as olive oil or ethanol. These solvents are just as effective at extracting CBD oil, but remove the risk of toxic residue.

However, natural solvent extraction is not without its downsides. When natural solvents like ethanol are used, chlorophyll may also be extracted. This gives the resulting oil an unpleasant taste. If the CBD is used in capsules or topicals, this isn't a big deal, but many CBD products are eaten or inhaled (such as gummies, tinctures, vape oils), so this can make them harder to sell.

The larger problem with natural solvents, though, is that they don't evaporate very well. As a result, the CBD extract contains a lower concentration of CBD than it would with other methods.

What Happens After Extraction?

After extraction, the resulting CBD oil is described as "full-spectrum." This means that other cannabinoids besides CBD, including CBDA, CBDV, THC, and others, are still present. As long as the product is sourced from hemp, the amount of THC will be 0.3% or less (which makes it legal anywhere in the U.S.).

Full-spectrum CBD oils also contain other beneficial elements from the plant material, such as terpenes and amino acids. Many people prefer full-spectrum CBD oil because of the "entourage effect." While this effect has not been proven, some users believe that the CBD is able to engage the endocannabinoid system more effectively when more cannabinoids are present.

However, some people would rather have no THC in their oil, even in very low, legal amounts. These people prefer CBD isolates. To create CBD isolate, the extract is cooled and further purified into crystalline isolate form. This results in a white, flavorless powder. Because it contains only CBD, CBD isolate is less expensive per milligram, contains no THC, and has no flavor or odor.

Finally, regardless of whether it is turned into a CBD isolate or remains full-spectrum, the CBD oil is added to other substances to create various CBD products.

The CBD may be mixed with a carrier oil like hemp seed oil or coconut oil to create CBD oil tinctures.

To create CBD gummies, the CBD oil may be combined with natural flavoring, juice, and organic corn syrup.

The CBD oil may be mixed with a variety of ingredients to create CBD edibles like baked goods or chocolates.

With CBD capsules, the CBD oil is often added to MCT oil (a coconut oil extract) to give the capsule volume. If it's a softgel, the capsule may also use olive oil to create the casing.

To create CBD vape oils, the CBD oil is combined with a mix of vegetable glycerin and propylene glycol (to make it suitable for inhalation) and natural flavoring (for better taste).

The CBD oil may be combined with various essential oils, shea butter, aloe vera, and waxes to create CBD creams, skin salves, and other topicals.

CBD OIL FOR FERTILITY

Women need better chances to conceive, and they must use something that will help them get pregnant. A woman who wants to make her body more likely to conceive should try CBD oil because it can do everything. These women will be amazed that they can use CBD oil to conceive, and they will find that they could improve their fertility simply by using these oils in a few different ways in their own food. CBD oil will help combats things that cause fertility to drop, and CBD oil could be the only thing that a woman needs in order to finally conceive.

CBD Oil Helps Reduce Anxiety And Depression

CBD oil bought at a place like American Hemp Oil helps women reduce anxiety and depression that could get in the way of fertility. A woman who is concerned about her fertility needs to take CBD tinctures every day, rub the oil on her belly, or use the oil in her smoothies or shakes to get their heartrate down. CBD oil helps women recover their energy so that their body can conceive much more easily.

CBD Oil Helps With Blood Flow

Women need as much blood flow as they can get if they plan to conceive, and that blood flow can be increased by little helpings of CBD oil. The tinctures will help women have better circulation, and that will help their heartrate remain lower. The combination of these two things makes it easier for a woman to conceive because she can have blood flowing and keep her body as relaxed as possible.

CBD Oil Helps with Pain

Women who live with chronic pain are often having a hard time conceiving because their body is focused on the chronic pain that they experience, and that pain can make it almost impossible for them to conceive. These women need to have a CBD oil tincture at least once a day, or they could use the oil on their bodies to help relieve the pain. The people that have the most pain are least likely to conceive because their body is much more focused on trying to get well. Because of this, a little CBD oil will go a long way in helping a woman have the baby she has hoped for her whole life.

Women who are using CBD oil will not have to worry about putting chemicals in their bodies that could hurt a baby if they do get pregnant. Women will often go the extra mile to make sure that their body is a safe environment for a child to grow, and they will use CBD oil because they know that it is safe and natural.

CBD oil is one of those things that women can use when they want to have a better chance of having a baby, and they can completely change how they approach pregnancy because they will have something that works in all situations. They can use it on their bodies, in their food, or take it for anxiety or depression. Helping with all these things makes it easier for a woman to get pregnant.

Infertility is something both men and women struggle with. So, does CBD oil help or hurt your chances at pregnancy?

CBD oil has been praised for its many potential health benefits and its use in the treatment of several chronic and acute conditions. However, despite CBD oil's growing popularity, there are still a number of unanswered questions like, does CBD oil affect fertility?

Currently, there's a lack of evidence to definitively state whether CBD oil has a positive or negative effect on human fertility. While products derived from cannabis are now legalized in most states, there are ethical implications of conducting tests on individuals who are trying to become pregnant. Because of this, we may not have a conclusive answer as to whether CBD oil impacts fertility for years to come.

While using CBD oil may indirectly help with conception-related issues that aren't physical in nature (e.g. sleep and mood), there are also studies that have shown CBD oil consumption could negatively affect fertility. In short, the jury's still out on whether using CBD oil could positively or negatively affect one's ability to get pregnant, which is why it's important to do as much research as possible on CBD oil and fertility before making a final decision.

Below, we'll go over what we currently know about CBD oil's potential benefits and risks as they apply to human fertility. With this information, you can decide on the best path forward for you and your partner.

CBD Oil and Fertility in People Without a Medical Explanation

For some people, conceiving is difficult for reasons that aren't purely medical. Sometimes there are lifestyle factors or mental roadblocks that get in the way of successful conception; in these cases, CBD oil may be able to help.

CBD Oil May Improve Fertility Through Sleep

Researchers believe there may be a correlation between insomnia and low fertility rates, with a studies suggesting the link is so strong that sleep disorders could be considered comorbid with both male and female infertility.

CBD oil can do a number of things to improve sleep quality, including regulating the production of catabolic hormones like cortisol. Cortisol is often referred to as a "stress hormone" because it is released when the body feels threatened by real or perceived danger. Cortisol can prevent the onset of sleep, or stop us from sleeping deeply, limiting the REM sleep that our body needs.

As an anti-catabolic supplement, CBD oil interferes with the secretion of cortisol, allowing for a better, deeper, and more restful sleep, according to a study performed at the University of San Paolo, Brazil. With this in mind, it's possible that CBD use could improve a person's sleep, thereby improving their chances of conceiving a child.

CBD Oil May Improve Fertility Through Mood

You may have heard about people with ongoing fertility struggles suddenly—and "miraculously"—conceiving successfully without much explanation as to why

Believe it or not, your mood and mental wellness can play an important role in pregnancy and fertility. Studies on both male and female test subjects have found links between poor mental health and decreased fertility rates, finding a possible correlation between stress, anxiety, and depression's effect on the release of hormones that regulate ovulation in women, and sperm production in men.

The role CBD oil can play in elevating a person's mood is due to its impact on a range of neurotransmitters, most notably anandamide and adenosine.

Anandamide is commonly called the "bliss molecule" and is responsible for feelings of joy, happiness, and motivation. CBD oil acts as an anandamide reuptake inhibitor, stopping the neurotransmitter from being reabsorbed and thus increasing the amount which is present in the brain, resulting in an improved and elevated mood.

CBD oil works similarly on the reuptake of adenosine. While this process is much less understood, it is believed that adenosine receptor A2A, when triggered, plays a role in anxiety and depression. By inhibiting the A2A receptor, mood is elevated and depressive symptoms are reduced.

While CBD oil may provide part of a solution to mood-induced fertility issues, there could still be a myriad of other factors at play affecting a person's ability to get pregnant.

How CBD Oil May Help with the Main Causes of Infertility

Two primary and manageable contributors to infertility are obesity and smoking. Luckily, CBD oil can help in reducing and ultimately putting an end to both of these afflictions.

CBD oil has been known to reduce addictive behaviors and can help people quit nicotine. CBD oil can also improve sleep, reduce stress and anxiety, and reduce the pain associated with working out—all risk factors for weight gain.

CBD Oil and Fertility: The Risks

Unfortunately, when it comes to fertility, CBD oil is not without its risks.

A number of studies conducted on animal test subjects have produced results that suggest CBD oil may actually inhibit fertility. One study on male mice found a 30% reduction in fertility rate in the group that had been treated with cannabidiol (CBD oil), while another trial of CBD on sea urchins found that "cannabinoids directly affect the process of fertilization in sea urchins by reducing the fertilizing capacity of sperm."

While there isn't a definitive correlation between these studies and the effects of CBD oil on humans' fertility, it's worth taking into account when considering your options.

CBD Oil and Fertility: The Jury's Still Out

Deciding whether or not to use CBD oil when trying to become pregnant is complicated.

While CBD oil is typically considered to be very safe, with the World Health Organization (WHO) stating CBD oil is generally well tolerated, more research is needed on the effects of CBD oil on fertility rates in humans, specifically.

At this point, it's best to speak to your doctor about all of your options when it comes to infertility treatments. Together you can decide if CBD oil is right for you and your family planning goals. You can also consult with a cannabis doctor who specializes in using cannabidiol as a medical treatment option.

CONCLUSION

You may already be aware that tetrahydrocannabinol (THC), the psychoactive compound in cannabis, activates certain receptors in the human endocannabinoid system, which determines the functioning of the internal reproductive organs, apart from regulating mood, hunger, etc.

A study involving 1,215 men — out of whom 130 individuals take cannabis more than once a week in the past 3 months — found that the subjects who smoked witnessed a 29% reduction in the total sperm count. However, the cells were the same size and shape and apparently had no difficulty swimming.

Also, in women, the drug is thought to delay or prevent ovulation. This can be corroborated from a study featuring 201 women — out of whom 29 individuals consumed canabis in the past 3 months — which found that smoking the drug seemed to put off ovulating for between 1.7 to 3.5 days on average.

Although the authors confirmed that smoking marijuana doesn't affect a person's ability to conceive, it may exacerbate already existing issues. To confirm the former inference, the group cited a U.S. survey that couldn't find any link between struggling to conceive and smoking weed for once a month to every day. However, for couples already dealing with infertility, the changes in sperm count and ovulatory function associated with smoking weed could further increase their difficulty in conceiving.

Scientists, however, agree that the aforesaid results may not be completely reliable considering the fact that people often shy away from telling the truth when it comes to illegal drugs, which are further plagued by the stigma the society has attached with them for centuries.

Delay in ovulation

A further reduced ability to conceive IF a couple is already dealing with the same

What cannabis doesn't seem to affect, include:

 The shape, size and swimming ability of the sperm cells

The ability to conceive in healthy couples

The use of cannabis may not bring about positive effects on fertility, but the good news is that it will not cause any permanent damage to a woman's ability to conceive.

 The only thing to remember is if you are having some trouble getting pregnant now, using cannabis possibly won't make things any easier for you or your partner. In other words, cannabis might slow things down for couples trying to get pregnant.

This means that you may have to put away the vape or skip rolling a joint while you try to conceive so that you can get your reproductive systems back in working order.

It is also worth noting that because of the illegal status of cannabis at federal level in the U.S., there really isn't enough concrete evidence to fully support the suggested adverse effects of cannabis on fertility. So we really cannot say for sure until more advanced research is done in humans (and not in mice or monkeys).

.